YOUR KNOWLEDGE HAS VALUE

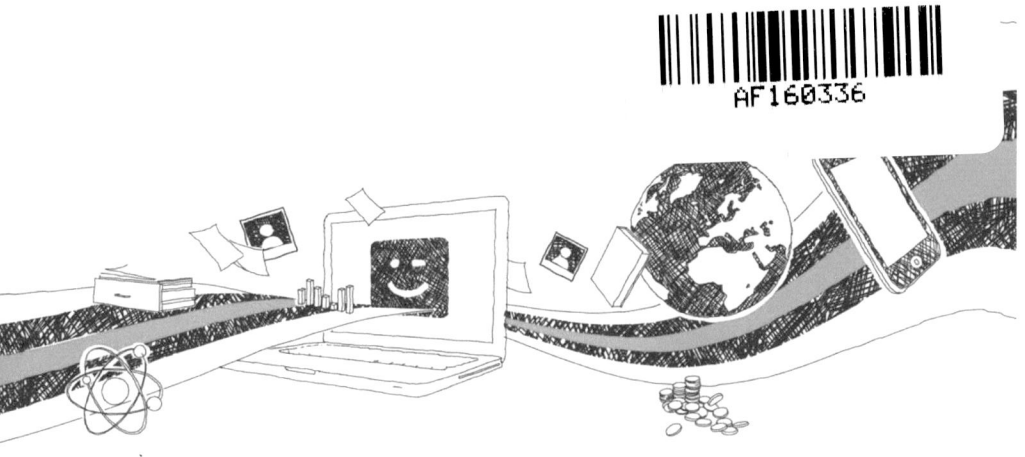

- We will publish your bachelor's and master's thesis, essays and papers

- Your own eBook and book - sold worldwide in all relevant shops

- Earn money with each sale

Upload your text at www.GRIN.com
and publish for free

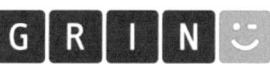

Bibliographic information published by the German National Library:

The German National Library lists this publication in the National Bibliography; detailed bibliographic data are available on the Internet at http://dnb.dnb.de .

This book is copyright material and must not be copied, reproduced, transferred, distributed, leased, licensed or publicly performed or used in any way except as specifically permitted in writing by the publishers, as allowed under the terms and conditions under which it was purchased or as strictly permitted by applicable copyright law. Any unauthorized distribution or use of this text may be a direct infringement of the author s and publisher s rights and those responsible may be liable in law accordingly.

Imprint:

Copyright © 2017 GRIN Verlag, Open Publishing GmbH
Print and binding: Books on Demand GmbH, Norderstedt Germany
ISBN: 9783668581746

This book at GRIN:

http://www.grin.com/en/e-book/381291/does-the-use-of-cell-phones-increase-the-risk-of-breast-cancer-an-investigation

Patrick Kimuyu

Does the Use of Cell Phones Increase the Risk of Breast Cancer? An Investigation

GRIN Publishing

GRIN - Your knowledge has value

Since its foundation in 1998, GRIN has specialized in publishing academic texts by students, college teachers and other academics as e-book and printed book. The website www.grin.com is an ideal platform for presenting term papers, final papers, scientific essays, dissertations and specialist books.

Visit us on the internet:

http://www.grin.com/

http://www.facebook.com/grincom

http://www.twitter.com/grin_com

Do Cell Phones Increase the Risk of Breast Cancer?

Name: Patrick K. Kimuyu

Breast cancer has been presenting diverse trends for decades and its increased prevalence in young women has raised concern among scientists. In practice, breast cancer is characterized by the growth of tumor cells in the breast tissue. Breast cancer is believed to have claimed many human lives in the past four decades, but its prevalence has decreased significantly due to improved disease awareness and treatment (Coltrera & Kaelin, 2005). Additionally, the observed decrease in cancer prevalence rate is also attributed to effective breast cancer screening that has enabled healthcare professionals to detect breast cancer cells at the early stages of the disease onset. Recent medical data show that about 230, 480 women in the U.S have invasive breast cancer. Further medical reports show that 57, 650 women have developed non-invasive breast cancer (Stoppler, 2016). Consequently, it is estimated that the prevalence rate of breast cancer has reached 13 percent, and this has made the number of breast cancer survivors in the U.S to reach 2.5 million individuals. Ductal breast cancer has been identified to be the most prevalent with a prevalence rate of 80% while lobular cancer comes second with 15% prevalence rate. Other types of breast cancers such as inflammatory breast cancer, medullary cancer and angiosarcoma account for 5% of all breast cancer cases (Ogden, 2004). Breast cancer is posing serious threats to women, although men have also been found to suffer from breast cancer. Therefore, this paper will provide an overview of breast cancer disease. It will also answer the research question: 'Does women carrying cell phones in their bras increase their chances of breast cancer, making breast cancer more frequent in younger women?'

Breast cancer begins as asymptomatic disease, but its signs and symptoms become conspicuous as the disease progresses. Ordinarily, abnormality on mammography is usually suspected to be caused by cancerous cells in the breast tissue. Additionally, development of persistent breast lump especially above the collarbone and the armpit serve as the principal signs of breast cancer (Stoppler, 2016). Other symptoms of breast cancer include nipple inversion and breast discharge, but intensive evaluation has to be conducted by a physician.

It has been found that breast cancer in women is caused by issues associated to age and gender, but there are no known etiological agents. Risk factors that are believed to be associated to breast cancers are usually categorized into three determinants: environmental factors, hormonal and reproductive factors, and family history factors (Stoppler, 2016). Recent epidemiologic analysis indicates that about 78 percent of breast cancer occurs in postmenopausal women. Further epidemiological studies show that about 73% of breast cancer in women is caused by environmental factors (Ogden, 2004).

Breast cancer diagnosis includes mammography, examination of the breast and ultrasonography. However, biopsy analysis serves as the definitive approach to diagnose breast cancer in women. Breast examination is conducted to identify the lump, and then mammograms help to define the nature of the breast lump. Ultrasound and MRI provide detailed information about conditions identified through mammography (Stoppler, 2016). Finally, histopathological investigations are carried out using breast tissue biopsy so as to identify cancerous cells.

Treatment of breast cancer consists of chemotherapy, surgery and radiation. Chemotherapy involves adjuvant chemotherapy and therapeutic chemotherapy, and this approaches aim at destroying cancer cells. On the other hand, Lumpectomy help to remove tumor cells through surgery while radiation involves directing radiation beams to the affected region so as to destroy cancerous cells (Stoppler, 2016).

In a general, breast cancer seems to be claiming the lives of women in the United States of America at an alarming rate. Therefore, efficient breast cancer management approaches are required so as to curb the problem. Some of the key approaches include public awareness, disease screening and treatment. The population requires vast understanding about predisposing risk factors, so as to be informed of the appropriate measures that will help reduce the prevalence of breast cancer among women (Ogden, 2004).

Owing to the link between breast cancer and cell phones use among young women who keep their cell phones in their bras, there seems to be immense controversy because there is no universal understanding among scientists. Some scientists maintain that, cell phone use do not have association with increased risk of cancer in humans while others refute such claims and support their stand with research findings.

Currently, the number of women carrying cell phones in their bras has increased significantly. That is, probably the principal reason as to why some scientist suggest the increasing trends of new cancer cases in young women is related to their cell phone storage. Johnson (2013) reports "millions of women, especially young ones, choose to keep their cell phone in their bra. It is convenient because it allows women to ditch their purse and remain hands-free" (par. 3). It has also been found out that most clothes worn by women do not have pockets, and this seems to be the reason, as to why they prefer storing their items in the purse including cell phones. However, the bra is as much convenient for cell phone storage as the purse, although it has some advantages over the purse. For instance, storing cell phones in bras enables women to continue receiving calls in noisy environments because it is easy to receive ringing alerts when the cell phone is in vibration mode. These are the principal reasons as to why "women carrying cell phones in their bras is becoming even more popular; in fact, bras with pockets for cell phones are now on the market" (Johnson, 2013, par. 9). In a recent survey conducted among college females, 40% of young women were found to be placing cell phones in their bras in which 3% of college females reported storing cell phones in brasseries for more than 10 hours a day (Johnson, 2013).

Over the past two decades, there have been concerns on the breast cancer risks caused by cell phones. Therefore, the principal question that everybody concerned should ask is why there is concern that cell phones may be increasing cancer risks among young women. Currently, the trends of new breast cancer cases among young women in the U.S are assuming upward trends unlike in the past when the rate of breast cancer in women aged below 34 years remained at 1.8% (SEER, 2014). In theory, there are several reasons as to why scientists are concerned with the health consequences of cell phones, especially with regard to breast cancer, which is presenting new trends among the U.S population and the world at large. Some of the main reasons include the emission of non-ionizing radiation, increase in cell phones among women and the length of cell phone storage in the bras. It is believed that cell phones emit non-ionizing radiation, which is referred to as radiofrequency energy. These radio waves are absorbed by the areas adjacent to the cell phone, although their absorption depends on the specific absorption rate (SAR) of a given cell phone. The second reason, as to why scientists have raised concern over the storage of cell phones in the bras of women is that the number of women with cell phones has increased significantly given that 303 million people in the United States were subscribed to cell phone services by 2010. This was a three-fold increase from 2000 in which the total number of cell phone subscribers was found to be 110 million. On the other hand, cell phone subscription has increased significantly around the globe since the invention of cell phones in which the total number of cell phone subscribers is estimated to be 5 billion. This reveals that a high percentage of women are exposed to breast cancer risk if at all there is any link between cell phones and breast cancer. Thirdly, scientists have raised concern over the matter because most women are extending the time they store cell phones in their bras to as high as 10 hours a day as it was reported in the survey conducted in college females. This is believed to increase the breast exposure to radiations. Ordinarily, low absorptions of radio waves from cell phones do not contain adequate energy to damage DNA molecules in the exposed body region (West et al., 2013). The American Cancer Society (2016) reports "at very high levels; RF waves can heat up body tissues, but the levels of energy given off by cell phones are much lower, and are not enough to raise temperatures in the body" (par. 4). Therefore, it is suggested that increased exposure of young women's' breasts to radio waves from cell phones stored in their bras may be causing DNA damage in the adjacent breast areas leading to the development of invasive tumors. It is believed that, these cell phone radiations may cause increased harm on the breast of young females compared to women aged 34 years and above because young breast exhibit diverse developmental feature such as high levels of metabolism and DNA replication for cellular growth.

Despite the revelations that cell phones may be increasing the risk of cancer, especially with regard to breast cancer in young women who have developed habits of storing their cell phones in bras, research studies on the issue of cell phones and cancer risks present controversial findings.

Currently, there is no evidence showing that radiofrequency energy emitted by cell phones causes cancer in humans nor is there evidence of cancer-causing effects on cells or laboratory animals. Ordinarily, ionizing radiations such as X-rays are known to cause cancer in humans through enhancing cancer-causing carcinogens which cause DNA damage, but non-ionizing radiations such as the radiofrequency energy produced by cell phones have not been found to be adequate for causing DNA damage (National Cancer Institute, 2016). In practice, DNA damage enhances the development of cancer; thus, low frequency radiations such as RF suggest the lack of epidemiological link between the increased incidence rates of breast cancer among young females who store cell phones in their bras.

In general, earlier research studies, which investigated the possible connection between cell phones and cancer, did not show any significant link between the two. These studies involved diverse research designs to investigate the issue extensively. In one of the research study which was referred to as a 'cohort study', a large group of research participants was investigated over a long period. Thereafter, the rates of tumors between the population that used cell phones and non-cell phone user were compared, although there were no significant differences between the two groups. On the other hand, a case-control study was also carried out to ascertain whether cell phones were related to cancer risks. For instance, "the international CEFALO study, which compared children who were diagnosed with brain cancer between ages 7 and 19 with similar children who were not, found no relationship between their cell phone use and risk for brain cancer" (National Cancer Institute, 2016, par. 19). The second case-control study, which was carried out in the U.S failed to demonstrate any correlation between cell phone use and cancer risk. Despite the different approaches adopted in these studies, the phenomenon remained uncertain; thus, prompting scientist to engage in intensive research findings. In the past two decades, several research studies have been conducted in which some of them have produced significant research results.

Some of the most significant research studies which are worth mentioning include the Interphone study, Danish cohort study and the U.K Million Women study. The Interphone study is believed to be the largest case-control study which has ever been conducted regarding the use of cell phones and cancer risks. This study comprised of clinical research experts from thirteen countries, and this consortium has been publishing analysis on the topic for some time. However, most of the published analyses do not indicate statistically significant association between cell phone use and cancer incidences. These include the recent research report from the group which "found no relationship between brain tumor locations and regions of the brain that were exposed to the highest level of radiofrequency energy from cell phones" (National Cancer Institute, 2016, par. 13).

The Danish cohort study included 358,000 Danish cell phone users who had brain tumors, in which Danish Cancer Registry was used as the principal source of information during the study. According to the National Cancer Institute (2016) report, the Danish cohort study "analyses found no association between cell phone use and the incidence of glioma, meningioma, or acoustic neuroma, even among people who had been cell phone subscribers for 13 or more years" (par. 14).

On the other hand, the prospective Million Women study, which was carried out in the United Kingdom showed that cell phone use does not have an association with increased cancer incidences. It was found out that cancer cases did not increase between 1998 and 2008 while cell phone subscribers increased rapidly over the same period. This revealed that there were no increased cancer risks caused by cell phone use among the study population. This research results has been reaffirmed by the research data obtained by the National Cancer Institute through the Surveillance, Epidemiology, and End Results (SEER) Program, which has compiled epidemiological data on cell phone use and cancer incidences between 1987 and 2007 (National Cancer Institute, 2016).

However, a research study report released in September 2013 provides evidence of the link between cell phones and breast cancer in young women. This research study was carried out by West et al. (2013), and it discovered breast cancer in four cases in which the patients who were aged between 21 to 39 years were reported to have been storing their cell phones in their bras. They report "a case series of four young women; ages from 21 to 39, with multifocal invasive breast cancer that raises the concern of a possible association with non-ionizing radiation of electromagnetic field exposures from cellular phones" (p. 1). They also report that, all the patients involved in the study "regularly carried their smart phones directly against their breasts in their brassieres for up to 10 hours a day, for several years, and developed tumors in areas of their breasts immediately underlying the phones" (p. 1). It is also reported that all the four women tested negative for BRCA2 and BRCA1 which investigates familial linkage of the disease. Therefore, it appeared evident that these young women lacked family history of breast cancer and they were reported to have no other cancer risk apart from their exposure to radiations from their cell phones. Moreover, these researchers report that reviews of the patients' breast imaging showed "showed clustering of multiple tumor foci in the breast directly under the area of phone contact" (West et al 1). On the other hand, pathology characteristics of the samples obtained from the four cases indicated similarities. One other most striking similarity noticed in the pathology reports is that, all tumors were found to be hormone-positive. Secondly, the tumors were found to be identical in morphology, and they showed extensive intraductal component. It was also noted that all the four tumors were of low-intermediate grade.

In regard to the case reports, the four cases investigated reveal the presence of a common etiological cause because they shared similarity in an array of pathological parameters. In case 1, a 21-year old female was reported to have been storing cell phone in the bra on the left side each day. This patient experienced spontaneous bloody nipple discharge and her mammogram indicated pleomorphic calcification in the retroareolar region. On the other hand, her pathology results showed extensive ductal carcinoma in situ (DCIS) which was found to be multifocal micro-invasive in nature (West et al 2).

Case 2 involved a 21-year old female who presented with a palpable breast mass. This mass was found in her left breast covering the area where she kept her cell phone, in which it was reported that she had been keeping the device in her bra for 6 years for at least 8 hours a day. Her mastectomy revealed extensive ductal carcinoma in situ in which two axillary lymph nodes in the left breast were found to be positive for metastatic disease, which had extended to the bone (West et al 2).

In case 3, a 33-year old female who had been storing cell phone in her bra on the right breast for 8 years was diagnosed with two palpable masses. Her mastectomy revealed extensive ductal carcinoma in situ with one sentinel lymph node being metastatic.

Finally, the fourth case involved a 39-year old female who had been placing her cell phone in contact with her right breast while using a Bluetooth device or communication for several hours a day during a ten-year span. She presented palpable masses, and her mastectomy indicated the presence of metastatic disease in two lymph nodes in the breast (West et al 2).

Despite the clinical relevancy provided by the four cases, these scientists caution "this series of four young women with cellular phone-related breast cancer is noteworthy, but caution must be exercised in drawing any conclusion from our small sample. Millions of women are using cellular devices, and it is predictable that rare events will occur" (West et al 3). They site reference of their conclusion, which compromises the validity of the cases on the small number of case series. West and his colleges state "From this small case series, one cannot infer causality but can only consider association; no data is available on the number of women who place their cellular phones in contact with their breast and do not develop breast cancer" (3). In addition, they state that the location of the placement of the cell phone and the duration of exposure are subject to recall bias. As a result, they remark "Cellular phone use continues to expand rapidly, especially among young adults. Until more data becomes available, efforts should be made to encourage cellular phone users to follow the recommendations of mobile device manufacturers and avoid skin contact" (West et al 3). From a medical perspective, they advise physicians to "document this behavior and also inform their patients that, until sufficient safety data becomes available, prolonged skin contact with cellular devices should be avoided" (West et al., 2013).

It is believed that, the lack of validity in the recently published analysis on the link between cell phones and breast cancer risk has created immense controversy and aroused unprecedented debate over the issue. For instance, Dr. Mehmet Oz, a research scientist introduced a new case of breast cancer, which he claims to be associated to a cell phone use. Shortly, after West and his colleagues published their reports in September 2013, Dr. Mehmet Oz claimed to have noticed breast cancer in Tiffany Frantz whom he claimed to have been storing her cell phone in contact with her breasts. As Gorski (2013) reports, Dr. Oz "believes that carrying her cell phone in her bra caused her cancer because it was on the same side and in the same area where her phone came into contact with her skin" (par. 7). This claim has sparked immense criticism from scientists who claim that Dr. Oz's report lacks scientific evidence. It is believed that Dr. Oz flouted research guidelines in his investigation. In addition, he reported a single case which is not based on existing literature regarding the issue.

Therefore, it is worth noting the conclusions made by expert agencies such as the International Agency for Research on Cancer (IARC), American Cancer Society (ACS), Center for Disease Control and Prevention, National Institute of Environmental Health

Sciences (NIEHS), Food and Drug Administration (FDA), and Federal Communications Commission (FCC). These agencies conclude that there is no scientific evidence that cell phones cause cancer, although extensive research in this area is still required for universal understanding. For instance, CDC states "scientific research as a whole does not support a statistically significant association between cell phone use and health effects" (National Cancer Institute, 2016, par. 32). In this respect, it is wise to conclude that cell phones are not associated to the increase of breast cancer in young women.

References

American Cancer Society (2016). *Cellular Phones*. Retrieved from http://www.cancer.org/cancer/cancercauses/othercarcinogens/athome/cellular-phones

Coltrera, F., & Kaelin, C. (2005). *Living through Breast Cancer: What a Harvard Doctor and Survivor Wants You to Know about Getting the Best Care While Preserving Your Self-Image*. New York, NY: McGraw-Hill.

Gorski, D. (2013). *"No, Carrying Your Cell Phone In Your Bra Will Not Cause Breast Cancer, No Matter What Dr. Oz Says*. Retrieved from http://sciencebasedmedicine.org/no-carrying-your-cell-phone-in-your-bra-will-not-cause-breast-cancer-no-matter-what-dr-oz-says/

Johnson, L. (2013, Dec. 27). Cancer Alert? Make Your Bra a 'No Phone Zone'. *CBN News*. Retrieved from http://www.cbn.com/cbnnews/healthscience/2013/December/Cancer-Alert-Make-Your-Bra-a-No-Phone-Zone/

National Cancer Institute (2016). *Cell Phones and Cancer Risk*. Retrieved from http://www.cancer.gov/cancertopics/factsheet/Risk/cellphones

Ogden, J. (2004). *Understanding Breast Cancer*, Hoboken, NJ: Wiley & Sons Ltd.

SEER (2014). *SEER Stat Fact Sheets: Breast Cancer*. Retrieved from http://seer.cancer.gov/statfacts/html/breast.html

Stoppler, M. (2016). *Breast Cancer*. Retrieved from http://www.emedicinehealth.com/breast_cancer/article_em.htm

West, J., Kapoor, N., Liao, S., Chen, J., Baily, L., & Nagourney, R. (2013). Multifocal Breast Cancer in Young Women with Prolonged Contact between their Breasts and their Cellular Phones. *Case Rep Med.*, *354682*, 1-4.

YOUR KNOWLEDGE HAS VALUE

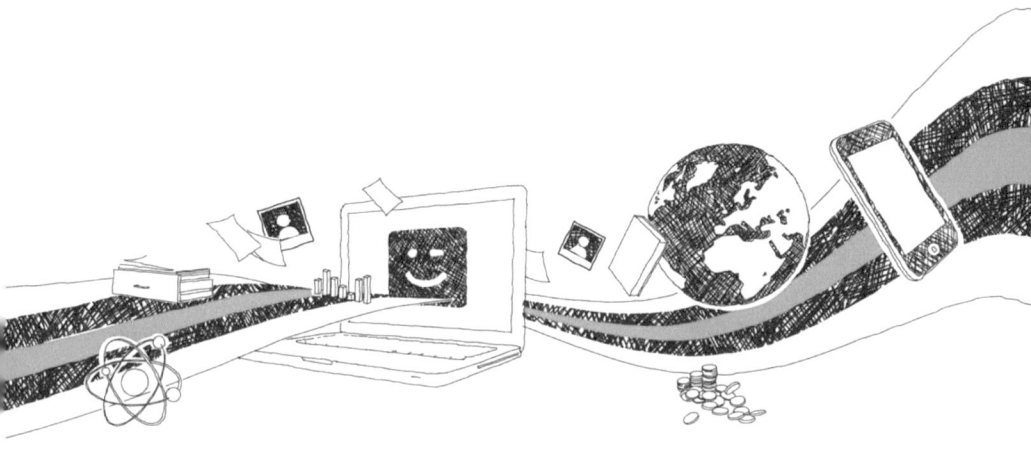

- We will publish your bachelor's and master's thesis, essays and papers

- Your own eBook and book - sold worldwide in all relevant shops

- Earn money with each sale

Upload your text at www.GRIN.com and publish for free

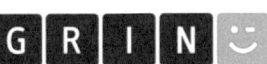